ELIMINATE FIBROIDS

Proven Methods To Eliminate, Prevent, and Shrink Fibroids Using The Latest Scientific Research

J. Olorun

This book contains the opinions and ideas of its author. It is intended to provide helpful general information on the subjects that it addresses. Neither the author nor publisher is engaged in rendering professional advice or services to the individual reader. The ideas, procedures, and suggestions contained in this book are not intended as a substitute for the advice of the reader's own physician(s) or other medical professionals based on the reader's own individual conditions, symptoms, or concerns. If the reader needs personal medical, health, dietary, exercise, or other assistance or advice, the reader should consult a competent physician and/or other qualified health care professionals. The author and publisher specifically disclaim all responsibility for injury, damage, or loss that the reader may incur as a direct or indirect consequence of following any directions or suggestions given in the book or participating in any activities described in the book.

ISBN-13: 9780578909233

This book may be purchased in bulk for promotional, educational or business use. Please contact J. Olorun at info@eliminatefibroids.com

To Doris Watson

CONTENTS

INTRODUCTION

This book is designed to provide the average person with the information necessary to feel comfortable and confident enough to tackle the challenges of living with fibroid tumors. This book provides the reader with only the essential information regarding the elimination, prevention, and reduction of fibroids. This book is meant to be a guide that will help combat the physical and emotional burden that accompanies living with fibroids. It provides all the information needed to design a personal action plan that will assist in eliminating, preventing, and shrinking fibroids, while subsequently reducing symptoms. This book provides the reader with the latest scientific research covering the elimination, prevention, and treatment of fibroids, compiled and condensed without any unwanted filler. The medical and scientific information in this book is presented so that it can be easily understood by the average person. This book should be used as a handbook to easily reference treatments, medical terms, and definitions relating to fibroids. It is recommended that this book is read both before and after visiting the gynecologist so that the reader is familiar with any medical terms, and treatments relating to fibroids.

HOW TO UTILIZE THIS BOOK

This book should be used as a functional and practical guide that you should read and reread in order to obtain a proper understanding of your condition along with it's specific medical terms and treatments. Use the diagrams in this book to become familiar with the various locations within the uterus that fibroids can form. Use the information in this book to familiarize yourself with the areas of your body as well as your organs that may be affected by the presence of fibroids. Use the 28 provided references to research articles cited within this book to conduct further detailed research into any specific study. Use this book's sections on medical, surgical, and alternative treatments to assist in determining your proper course of action. Use the mental preparation information provided in this book to assist in overcoming the mental hurdles of having fibroids. If planning to have a child, use this book's section on pregnancy and fibroids to help plan your pregnancy. Lastly, use this book's important questions for the doctor section to help gather as much important information as possible from your doctor regarding your condition.

WHAT ARE FIBROIDS?

Uterine fibroids are non cancerous benign fibrous tumors comprised of smooth muscle tissue that are found in many women during their reproductive years. Their size ranges from as small as a seed to as large as a melon. Women between the ages of 18-45 are most likely to develop fibroids. The causes of uterine fibroids are currently unknown. However, there are several risk factors that are linked to their development and growth. Uterine fibroids are treated either medically or surgically.

The clinical name for fibroid is leiomyoma. Uterine leiomyomas (fibroids) are located within the uterus. The uterus is where a baby develops and grows during a woman's pregnancy. The uterus is located within the pelvic region. The pelvic region is located between the abdomen and thighs. Internally, the uterus is directly behind and almost overlying the bladder, and in front of the part of the large intestine that is closest to the rectum and anus. The size of the uterus is about 3 inches (7.6 cm) long, 1.8 inches (4.5 cm) wide, and 1.2 inches (3.0 cm) thick. The lower portion of the uterus is called the cervix. The cervix and cervical canal protrude into the vagina.

Location Of Uterus Within The Body

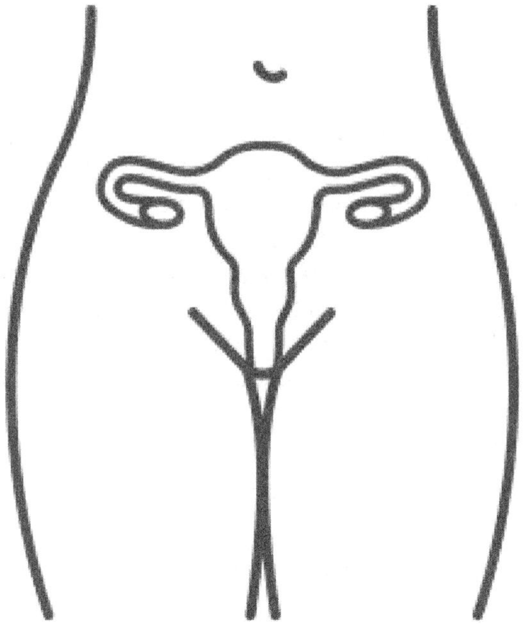

Fibroid Location Classifications

Uterine fibroids are located either within the wall of the uterus, the surface of the uterus, within the muscle beneath the wall of the uterus, or within the wall of the cervix. When located within the wall of the uterus they are referred to as **intramural fibroids**. When located on the surface of the uterus they are referred to as **subserosal fibroids**. When located within the muscle underneath the wall of the uterus they are referred to as **submucosal fibroids**. When located within the wall of the cervix they are referred to as **cervical/cervix fibroids**. When located on the outer surface of the uterus and are attached by a narrow stalk they are referred to as **pedunculated fibroids.** Fibroids can be single or multiple and their size varies from a few millimeters to 11.8 inches (30 cm) or more.

Fibroid Location Classifications

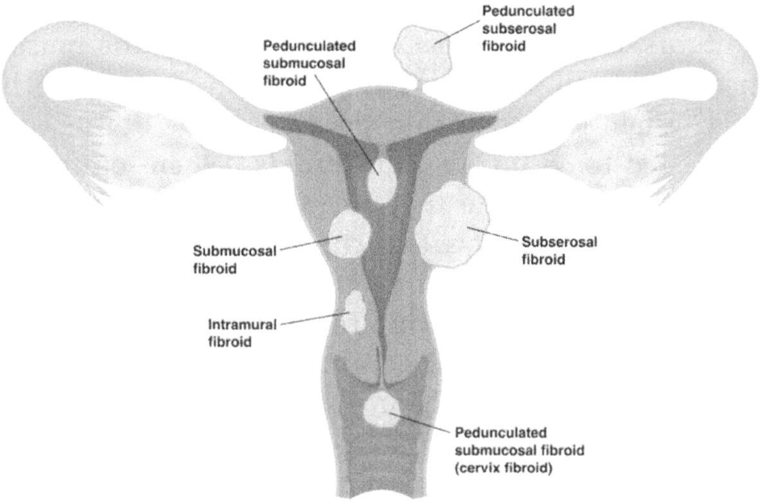

Symptoms

Symptoms associated with uterine fibroids include, heavy menstrual bleeding, anemia, pelvic pain, painful menstrual cramps, enlarged or distorted abdomen, pelvic pressure or discomfort, urinary tract problems such as frequency, urgency, and urinary incontinence; swelling of the kidney, bowel problems, constipation, and pain during sexual intercourse. However, some women with uterine fibroids do not display any symptoms. The location of the fibroid will affect the type of complications and symptoms experienced.

Specific symptoms and complications associated with fibroid location:

Subserosal: Often will become **pedunculated** (grow like a stalk); can cause severe pain if the fibroid wraps around stalk or the stalk becomes twisted and decreases blood supply.

Submucosal: Often will cause heavy bleeding; can cause the uterus lining to break causing severe bleeding; can cause leucorrhea (white or yellow discharge from the vagina).

Cervical/Cervix: Often causes heavy bleeding; can become infected; can cause leucorrhea (white or yellow discharge from the vagina).

Intramural: Can cause tilting of the cervix and uterus; can cause menstrual pain; can cause heavy bleeding during and between menstrual cycles; can cause back pain; can cause pelvic pain; can cause anemia (iron deficiency) due to blood loss.

Risk Factors

Risk factors include heredity, weight, and age. Heredity risk is higher in women with first degree relatives who have fibroids such as their parents and siblings. The incidence of uterine fibroids increases with age during the reproductive years of age 12 to 51. Weight gain and body fat also increases the risk of uterine fibroids.

By age 50 nearly 70% of white women and more than 80% of black women have developed at least one uterine fibroid. Black women tend to have larger fibroids that grow more quickly and are diagnosed at younger ages than white women. It is currently unclear why fibroids are more common in black women.

Cause

The cause of uterine fibroids is unknown, but genetic predispositions, prenatal hormone exposure, and the effects of hormones, have shown to cause the growth of fibroids. It is believed that the hormones estrogen and progesterone along with other hormones have a direct effect on fibroid cells. Estrogen is believed to promote the growth of uterine fibroids by influencing (directly and indirectly) a large number of proteins that stimulate cell growth. In Contrast, progesterone's influence on these proteins is believed to counteract the growth of uterine fibroids.

Diagnosis

Uterine fibroids are diagnosed after the completion of a pelvic examination during a routine visit to the gynecologist. Further examination with ultrasound scanning is completed in order to determine the size, location, and number of uterine fibroids. In some cases magnetic resonance imaging (MRI) is required to provide enhanced visualization of fibroids. Also, in some cases a procedure called a hysteroscopy may be performed. This is a surgical procedure where a telescope is inserted into the cavity of the uterus in order to determine the location of the fibroids.

Summary

Location: within the uterus

Size: can be as small as a seed to as large as a melon

Fibroid uterus location classifications: intramural, subserosal, submucosal, cervical, pedunculated

Common Symptoms: heavy bleeding, pelvic pain, distorted abdomen, constipation

Risk factors: heredity, age, weight

Cause: unknown, estrogen is believed to promote growth

Diagnosis methods: pelvic examination, ultrasound, MRI, hysteroscopy

MEDICAL TREATMENTS

Tranexamic acid/mefenamic acid is used to treat heavy bleeding and pain during menstrual cycles. It is a combination of two medicines: Tranexamic acid and mefenamic acid. Tranexamic acid is an anti-fibrinolytic. It works by preventing the breakdown of blood clots to control excessive bleeding during menstrual cycles. Mefenamic acid is a non-steroidal anti-inflammatory drug (NSAID) which blocks the production of certain chemical messengers (prostaglandins) that cause pain and inflammation (redness and swelling). The treatment involves taking tranexamic acid/mefenamic acid tablets.

Levonorgestrel releasing intrauterine system is a plastic device that is placed in the uterus where it slowly releases the hormone levonorgestrel. It reduces menstrual bleeding by thinning the lining of the uterus.

Ulipristal Acetate is a selective progesterone receptor modulator. It's used to shrink fibroids and reduce bleeding. The treatment involves taking one pill per day for 13 weeks.

Mifepristone is an antiestrogen hormone used to reduce

bleeding and pressure symptoms for up to six months. The treatment involves taking mifepristone tablets.

Gonadotropin releasing hormone agonists shrink fibroids and reduce bleeding by lowering estrogen levels. Treatment can only be given for a maximum of six months. The treatments are given in the form of injections.

SURGICAL TREATMENTS

Uterine **artery embolization** is a surgical procedure performed under local anesthesia. A thin catheter is inserted into the artery at either the groin or wrist. The incision is roughly the size of the tip of a pencil. Small particles are injected into the blood vessels that supply the uterus. This results in blockage of the blood supply to the fibroids and the fibroid begins to soften, bleed less, and shrink in size.

A **myomectomy** is a surgical procedure that's performed under general anesthesia to remove uterine fibroids. It involves making an incision through the skin on the lower abdomen and removing the fibroids from the wall of the uterus. The uterine muscle is then sewn back together using several layers of stitches.

A **hysterectomy** is a surgical procedure that's performed under general anesthesia to remove the uterus. It involves the surgeon making either a vertical incision from the navel to the pubic hairline or a horizontal incision made directly above the pubic hairline in order to remove the entire uterus.

MRI-guided focused ultrasound is a non-invasive procedure that uses a MRI scanner to send pulses of high power ultrasound targeted at fibroids through the skin of the lower abdomen.

Medical And Surgical Treatment Pros And Cons

Before determining a treatment option, it's important to consider the pros and cons of each option.

Medical Treatment Pros And Cons

Tranexamic acid/Mefenamic acid :
Pros: Reduces the amount of bleeding and pain associated with menstrual cycles.
Cons: Effectiveness for women with fibroids is uncertain.

Levonorgestrel releasing intrauterine system:
Pros: Reduces the amount of menstrual bleeding as well as provide contraception.
Cons: Not suitable for women with large fibroids.

Ulipristal Acetate:
Pros: Reduces the amount of menstrual bleeding and shrinks fibroids; does not cause menopausal side effect or bone loss.
Cons: Can cause irregular bleeding in women with submucosal fibroids; may be associated with liver toxicity; less successful in women with multiple or large fibroids.

Mifepristone:
Pros: Reduces bleeding and pressure symptoms for up to six months.
Cons: Does not shrink fibroids.

Gonadotropin releasing hormone agonists:
Pros: Can be used for 3-6 months presurgery to reduce fibroid size, and perioperative blood loss; helps correct iron deficiency anemia.
Cons: Can only be used for up to 6 months; given in the form of injections.

Surgical Treatments Pros And Cons

Uterine Artery Embolization:
Pros: Performed under local anesthesia; decreases fibroid size and menstrual blood loss; conserves uterus.
Cons: Improvement of symptoms can take up to six months.

Myomectomy:
Pros: Conserves uterus; removes fibroids; smaller incision than hysterectomy.
Cons: Possible recurrence of fibroids.

Hysterectomy:
Pros: Permanently removes fibroid symptoms.
Cons: Removes uterus; not suitable for women wanting to have children.

MRI-guided focused ultrasound:
Pros: Noninvasive, allows quicker return to normal

activities.

Cons: Not effective for several fibroids or very large fibroids.

Summary

Medical treatments:

Tranexamic acid/mefenamic acid
Levonorgestrel releasing intrauterine system
Ulipristal Acetate
Mifepristone
Gonadotropin releasing hormone agonists

Surgical treatments:

Uterine artery embolization
Myomectomy
Hysterectomy
MRI-guided focused ultrasound

ALTERNATIVE TREATMENTS

There are also non medical and non surgical treatment options that should be considered.

Dietary Solutions

The more information you obtain about fibroids as well as proper nutrition, the better equipped you'll be to take an active role in your health. A healthy diet that provides the proper nutrition will provide you with the foundation needed to live a disease free and healthy life.

The cause of uterine fibroids is unknown, but the hormone estrogen is believed to promote the growth of uterine fibroids. Estrogen is a hormone that is responsible for the development and regulation of the female reproductive system along with female sexual characteristics. Estrogen levels fall after menopause.

Subsequently, fibroids often shrink in size after entering

menopause as a result of the fall in the levels of the hormone estrogen. The average age of menopause is 51. Researchers have found that estrogen promotes the growth of uterine fibroids by influencing (directly and indirectly) a large number of proteins that stimulate cell growth.[1] Therefore, lowering estrogen levels may be a solution in inhibiting the growth of uterine fibroids. Consequently, there is scientific evidence that diet can influence the plasma level and excretion of estrogen.[2] There is also scientific evidence which shows that diet can influence the growth of uterine fibroids.[3, 4] Surprisingly, the diet shown to influence the plasma level and excretion of estrogen is similar to the diet shown to influence the growth of uterine fibroids. Both diets were considered vegetarian or plant based diets.

Scientific evidence that a vegetarian diet influences the plasma level and excretion of estrogen has been shown. Researchers studied vegetarian and non vegetarian premenopausal women and measured their estrogen levels and fecal samples. They found a positive correlation between fecal matter weight and fecal excretion of estrogen in both groups. They found that vegetarians had higher fecal weight and increased fecal excretion of estrogen.[2] The study concluded that vegetarian women had an increased fecal output, which lead to increased fecal excretion and a lower plasma level of estrogen.

Scientific evidence that a vegetarian diet has been shown to influence the growth of uterine fibroids has also been presented. Researchers studied 1200 women between the ages 30 and 50. The results concluded that a vegetarian diet correlated with a reduced risk of uterine fibroids. It was found that greater intake of fresh fruits and cruciferous vegetables may be able to reduce the incidence of uterine fibroids.[3]

Similarly, scientific evidence was presented that showed higher intake of green vegetables and fruits were associated with a lower risk of uterine fibroids.[5] Also, a scientific study conducted on Italian women showed that higher intake of meat and fish resulted in a greater risk of uterine fibroids.[5]

The Diet That Promotes Estrogen Excretion And Reduces The Prevalence Of Fibroids

A plant based diet is the best dietary option for removing excess estrogen from the body as well as reducing the overall risk of developing uterine fibroids. A plant based diet is a diet high in fruits, vegetables, and whole grain consumption, but low in meat consumption. These diets are typically referred to as vegetarian and vegan, eating no meat but eating dairy, or eating no meat as well as no dairy. A plant based diet is high in fiber and has shown to increase both fecal volume and frequency of defecation.[4,6] It has been shown scientifically that increased fecal matter weight is correlated with increased fecal excretion of estrogen. Consequently, vegetarians eating a plant based diet had higher fecal weight and increased fecal excretion of estrogen than meat eaters.[2] Thus, it was also found that a vegetarian diet resulted in a reduced risk of uterine fibroids.

Fiber

Fiber is the part of plant-based food (grains, fruits, vegetables, nuts, and beans) that the body can't digest or absorb. It passes relatively intact through the stomach, small intestine, and colon flushing toxins out of the body. Fiber normalizes bowel movements by increasing the weight and size of stools making them easier to pass. Thus, a high fiber diet will aid in the removal of excess estrogen. In turn, the removal of excess estrogen is beneficial in limiting the growth of fibroids.

Methods Of Increasing Fiber Intake:

Increase overall consumption of fruits, vegetables, and whole grains.

Make the first meal of the day a high fiber food.

Substitute white rice, white bread, and pasta with brown rice, whole wheat bread, and whole wheat pasta.

Substitute dessert with fruit.

Eat a salad with dinner.

Foods High In Fiber: Data From The U. S. Department Of Agriculture

High Fiber Fruits:
Avocado 9.2 grams (One peeled avocado)
Pear 5.5 grams (One medium pear)

Apple 5.4 grams (One large apple)
Prunes 3.4 grams (Five prunes)
Orange 3.4 grams (One orange)
Banana 3.1 grams (One medium banana)

High Fiber Vegetables:
Artichoke 6.9 grams (One medium artichoke)
Potato 6.3 grams (One large baked potato)
Sweet Potato 5.9 grams (One large baked sweet potato)
Winter Squash 5.7 grams (One cup)
Broccoli 5.1 grams (One cup)
Pumpkin 7.1 grams (One cup canned)

High Fiber Legumes:
Navy Beans 10.5 grams (Per100 grams)
Pinto Beans 9 grams (Per 100 grams)
Black Beans 8.7 grams (Per 100 grams)
Split Peas 8.3 grams (Per 100 grams)
Lentils 7.9 grams (Per 100 grams)
Lima Beans 7 grams (Per 100 grams)
Chickpeas 6.4 grams (Per 100 grams)
Kidney Beans 6.4 grams (Per 100 grams)

High Fiber Whole Grains:
Kamut 7.4 grams (One cup)
Spelt Pasta 5.5 grams (One cup)
Quinoa 5.1 grams (One cup)
Whole Wheat Pasta 11.8 grams (One cup)
Corn 3 grams (One cup)
Oats 8.1 grams (One cup)
Brown Rice 4 grams (One cup cooked)
Wild Rice 3 grams (One cup cooked)

The Fibroid Diet Plan

Eat a diet high in vegetables, fruits, whole grains, and beans. Avoid or eat less animal protein.

Foods to eat:
Cruciferous vegetables such as broccoli, cabbage cauliflower, collard greens, kale, and arugula.

A variety of fruits.

Whole grains.

Potassium rich foods such as bananas, tomatoes and sweet potatoes.

Beans.

Foods to avoid:
Animal protein and animal fats. (chicken ,beef, fish, turkey etc.)

Excess salt and sugar. (both causes the body to retain water and waste)

Soda and sugary drinks.

Caffeine.

Dairy. (milk and cheese)

Alcohol.

Nutritional Supplements

There is scientific evidence that certain nutritional supplements may also support in the reduction of a woman's risk in getting fibroids. Turmeric (Curcumin), vitamin D, and green tea extract have all shown to reduce the occurrence of fibroids.

Turmeric (Curcumin)

Curcumin, an ingredient in the spice turmeric, was found to inhibit the growth of uterine fibroid cells.[7, 8] Researchers took tissue samples of uterine fibroids and applied curcumin to them. The results showed that curcumin inhibited the growth of the uterine fibroid cells.[8]

Additional Benefits

Curcumim has also been shown to be effective in treating:

1. Arthritis [9, 10]
2. Lupus [11]
3. Lung disease [12]
4. Colon cancer [13]

Vitamin D

Similarly, vitamin D was also found to inhibit the growth of uterine fibroid cells. Tissue samples were obtained from women with uterine fibroids, the application of vitamin D to their samples inhibited the growth of uterine fibroid cells.[14] Researchers also found that an adequate amount of vitamin D is associated with a reduced risk of uterine fibroids.[14, 15] Researchers obtained blood samples from 1036 women. After testing their vitamin D levels it was determined that women with sufficient vitamin D levels had an estimated 32% reduced chance of having uterine fibroids.[15] The Institute of Medicine recommends 800 IU of vitamin D per day for adults.

Additional Benefits

Vitamin D has been shown to reduce the risk of:

1. Multiple sclerosis [16]
2. Heat disease [17]
3. Influenza [18]

Green Tea Extract

Epigallocatechin gallate (EGCG), the major ingredient in green tea has been shown to shrink uterine fibroids.[7, 11] Researchers conducted a 4 month study consisting of 33 women with uterine fibroids, of the 33 women, 22 women were given a treatment consisting of a daily dosage of 800 mg of green tea extract. The remaining 11 women were given a placebo and were unaware that they were not actually receiving any treatment. The results showed that their fibroid volume increased 24 % over the 4 month study period. However, the group of women actually given the treatment of green tea extract showed a decrease in fibroid volume of 32.6 % over the same 4 month study period.[19]

Additional Benefits

EGCG has also been shown to be effective in preventing:

1. Heart disease [20]
2. Diabetes [20]
3. Inflammation [20]

Summary

Alternative treatments:

High fiber diet with little to no animal protein nor animal fat.

Turmeric (Curcumin)

Vitamin D

Green Tea Extract (EGCG)

THINGS TO AVOID

Do not use an herbal douche or insert any herbs vaginally as a means of treating uterine fibroids. There have been examples of women experiencing severe internal damage as a result of vaginally inserted herbs used as a means of uterine fibroid treatment.[21]

Avoid eating a diet high in processed foods, red meats, and high fats. Such diets have shown to contribute to the growth of uterine fibroids as well as have an association of increased risk of uterine fibroids.[5, 22, 23]

Lastly, avoid taking a negative mental approach. Avoid focusing on the negative aspects of having fibroids.

THE PROPER MENTAL APPROACH

The experience of having uterine fibroids not only creates negative physical symptoms but also creates negative psychological symptoms. Therefore, it's important to embrace a positive mindset. Dealing with the negative symptoms of uterine fibroids over a long period of time often comes with a psychological cost. One may experience feelings of anger, frustration, fear, and depression. One may also experience denial. Denial is a refusal to accept reality. Often a person with uterine fibroids that is experiencing denial will deny that the fibroids exist because the idea of having fibroids is uncomfortable or disturbing. These negative emotional reactions usually result in the delay of treatment or the unwillingness to get treatment. Therefore, it's important for an individual to practice a positive mental approach in order to properly treat the condition as well as maintain and improve one's emotional well being.

People have a tendency to only focus on the negative and ignore the positive. However, this can be changed by intentionally trying to focus on the positive. A change in perspective from looking at the negative to focusing on any positive will combat feelings of sadness, anger, and fear. It has been found that a positive mental approach can lead to improved physical health.[24, 25, 26] It has also been found that individuals that focus on the positive aspects of things live a longer and healthier life.[27] Therefore, focusing on the positive such as a treatment option that will reduce or eliminate your symptoms will assist in combating the negative feelings that often result in despair and an unwillingness to seek treatment. Coincidentally, exercise has been shown to benefit feelings of well being and is also associated with less incidence of fibroids.[28] So always try to make an effort to maintain an optimistic outlook regarding your condition. It will benefit your overall health and happiness.

Summary

Never insert herbs vaginally.
Avoid eating a diet high in processed foods, red meats, and fats.
Embrace a positive mindset.
Focus on the positive.

ACTION PLAN

First and foremost, familiarize yourself with the information outlined within this book. Familiarize yourself with the common symptoms and complications of uterine fibroids. If you believe that you are experiencing symptoms of uterine fibroids schedule an examination with a gynecologist. If diagnosed with fibroids, familiarize yourself with all available treatment options. Try to maintain a positive mental outlook. Use the information in this book along with your gynecologist's recommendation to decide on a course of treatment. Your goal is to take an active role in the elimination, prevention, and treatment of fibroid tumors. Therefore, use the information in this book to start a diet plan that will immediately assist in reducing the accumulation of estrogen within your body.

A proper diet for fibroids will assist in the prevention and the reduction of fibroids. It's important to ensure that you do not experience constipation but instead have regular and frequent bowel movements. Having at least one bowel movement per day is considered frequent. Frequent bowel movements are important to assist the body in eliminating excess estrogen and waste. Subsequently, dairy products such as milk and cheese not only contribute to constipation but they also contribute to elevated estrogen levels within the body. Therefore, in order to prevent constipation as well as combat the accumulation of excess estrogen in the body, it is necessary to limit your consumption of dairy products. Either Almond milk or Rice milk can be used as a substitute for regular cow's milk.

Also, avoid eating a diet high in processed foods, red meats, and high fats. Eat a diet high in fruits, vegetables, and whole grains but low in meat and dairy consumption. Also, drink an adequate amount of water daily. Sufficient daily water intake will help prevent constipation along with assist the body in eliminating waste and excess estrogen. A half ounce of water per pound of body weight is considered an adequate amount of water for daily intake. Further examine the scientific research provided regarding the use of vitamin D, green tea extract, and turmeric and consider adding them to your daily regime as a means of combating fibroids. Lastly, remember to keep in good spirits and try to maintain a positive mental attitude.

When considering surgical or medical treatment options to eliminate your fibroids, understand that depending on the treatment option there may be a chance of recurrence. Therefore, in order to assist in preventing the recurrence of fibroids it's important to implement the fibroid diet plan immediately after your procedure. Immediately start a diet high in fiber that consists of a higher consumption of fruits, vegetables and whole grains while limiting dairy and meat intake. This will assist your body in alleviating any excess estrogen and help prevent the recurrence of fibroids.

Also, be mindful that fibroids will usually stop growing and accumulating after the onset of menopause. Menopause is when a woman's menstrual cycle stops permanently. Menopause generally starts between the ages of 40 and 50. This is usually accompanied by a reduction of estrogen which in turn results in the halting of the growth and accumulation of fibroids. Existing fibroids may also reduce slightly in size after the onset of menopause. Lastly, keep in mind that most birth control pills are high in estrogen and may subsequently contribute to the growth of uterine fibroids.

PREGNANCY AND FIBROIDS

If considering pregnancy, it is important to remember that the size, number, and location of fibroids will determine the proper course of action. Having a few small fibroids is usually no cause for concern. However, having large or multiple fibroids may pose a risk for pregnant women. Knowing the position and size of the fibroids will help you and your physician determine the proper course of action. If you are planning to have a child and you're diagnosed with fibroids, it's important to not get discouraged. Work with your doctor to ensure a healthy pregnancy and safe delivery of your baby. Some pregnancy related risks include:

Breech position: The baby may be breech if the fibroids are limiting space within the uterus. The breech position is a bottom down instead of head down position. If your physician determines the baby is not in the head down position they may recommend a cesarean section (c-section) delivery.

Incomplete cervical dilation: Fibroids limiting space in the lower portion of the uterus can block the opening of the birth canal. This can increase the risk of needing a c-section delivery.

Preterm delivery: Fibroids may stress the uterus; pain from fibroids may lead to preterm contractions which can result in an early delivery.

Abnormal placenta: Fibroids may cause the implantation of the placenta over the cervix or cause the placenta to break away from the uterine wall.

Poor contraction: Fibroids may cause the disruption of normal uterine tissue resulting in weak contractions. This can increase the risk of needing a c-section delivery.

Postpartum hemorrhage: Poor contractions due to fibroids can lead to bleeding after delivery. If the uterus cannot contract, uterine blood vessels may continue to bleed after delivery. Postpartum hemorrhage usually occurs within 24 to 48 hours after delivery and is considered a medical emergency.

IMPORTANT QUESTIONS FOR THE DOCTOR

It's important that while visiting your gynecologist that you feel comfortable asking any and all questions you have regarding your condition. It's common for people to feel intimidated by the doctor. However, it's important that you have your doctor explain all the necessary details of your condition as well as answer all of your questions so that you have a clear and complete understanding. Furthermore, if there is anything that the doctor tells you that you do not clearly understand, be sure to make the doctor aware that you are unclear and ask your doctor to explain it again with greater detail.

Questions To Ask The Gynecologist:

How Many Fibroids Do I Have?

Rationale/Reason for asking: The number of fibroids is a

factor in determining the proper treatment option.

What Are Their Sizes?

Rationale/Reason for asking: Very large fibroids are known to be associated with a higher rate of miscarriage, and preterm delivery. Some large fibroids may cause problems during delivery. Small fibroids that are not causing symptoms usually do not require treatment.
The size of the fibroids will also assist in determining the proper treatment option.

Where Are They Located?

Rationale/Reason for asking: Fibroids may push against the bladder or intestines causing digestive issues. Submucosal fibroids are known to be associated with a higher rate of miscarriage, and preterm delivery. The location will also assist in determining the proper treatment option.

What Are The Doctor's Recommendations And What Are The Pros And Cons Of Their Recommendations?

Rationale/Reason for asking: After familiarizing yourself with the information you've obtained regarding treatment pros and cons you will want to get your doctor's expert opinion.

Are There Any Other Recommendable Treatment Options Available And If So,

What Are The Pros And Cons?

Rationale/Reason for asking: You want to be well informed about all of the options available for treatment.

CONCLUSION

Start your journey to eliminating, preventing, and shrinking fibroids by familiarizing yourself with the common symptoms and complications of uterine fibroids. Become familiar with all available treatment options. Be sure to ask your doctor any and all questions you may have regarding your condition. Also, make sure you have a clear understanding of all the information provided by your doctor. It's important to maintain a positive mental outlook. It's also necessary to immediately start a diet plan that will assist in reducing the accumulation of estrogen within your body. Most importantly, always take an active role in improving your health. Finally, use the information contained within this book to rid you of the many hardships of living with fibroids.

EVIDENCE BASED RESEARCH

Use the following references to conduct more in-depth study.

1.Maruo, T. (2004). Sex steroidal regulation of uterine leiomyoma growth and apoptosis. *Human Reproduction Update, 10*(3), 207-20. https://doi.org/10.1093/humupd/dmh019

2.Goldin, B. R., Adlercreutz, H., Gorbach, S. L., Warram, J. H., Dwyer, J. T., Swenson, L., & Woods, M. N. (1982). Estrogen excretion patterns and plasma levels in vegetarian and omnivorous women. *New England Journal of Medicine, 307*(25), 1542-1547. https://doi.org/10.1056/nejm198212163072502

3.Shen, Y., Wu, Y., Lu, Q., & Ren, M. (2015). Vegetarian diet and reduced uterine fibroids risk: A case-control study in Nanjing, China. *Journal of Obstetrics and Gynaecology Research, 42*(1), 87-94. https://doi.org/10.1111/jog.12834

4.Yang, J. (2012). Effect of dietary fiber on constipation:

A meta analysis. *World Journal of Gastroenterology, 18*(48), 7378. https://doi.org/10.3748/wjg.v18.i48.7378

5.Parazzini, F., Di Martino, M., Candiani, M., & Viganò, P. (2015). Dietary components and uterine Leiomyomas: A review of published data. *Nutrition and Cancer, 67*(4), 569-579. https://doi.org/10.1080/01635581.2015.1015746

6.Davies, G. J., Crowder, M., Reid, B., & Dickerson, J. W. (1986). Bowel function measurements of individuals with different eating patterns. *Gut, 27*(2), 164-169. https://doi.org/10.1136/gut.27.2.164

7.Islam, M. S., Akhtar, M. M., Ciavattini, A., Giannubilo, S. R., Protic, O., Janjusevic, M., Procopio, A. D., Segars, J. H., Castellucci, M., & Ciarmela, P. (2014). Use of dietary phytochemicals to target inflammation, fibrosis, proliferation, and angiogenesis in uterine tissues: Promising options for prevention and treatment of uterine fibroids? *Molecular Nutrition & Food Research, 58*(8), 1667-1684. https://doi.org/10.1002/mnfr.201400134

8.Malik, M., Mendoza, M., Payson, M., & Catherino, W. H. (2009). Curcumin, a nutritional supplement with antineoplastic activity, enhances leiomyoma cell apoptosis and decreases fibronectin expression. *Fertility and Sterility, 91*(5), 2177-2184. https://doi.org/10.1016/j.fertnstert.2008.03.045

9.Chandran, B., & Goel, A. (2012). A randomized, pilot study to assess the efficacy and safety of curcumin in patients with active rheumatoid arthritis. *Phytotherapy*

Research, *26*(11), 1719-1725. https://doi.org/10.1002/ptr.4639

10.Kuptniratsaikul, V., Dajpratham, P., Taechaarpornkul, W., Buntragulpoontawee, M., Lukkanapichonchut, P., Chootip, C., Saengsuwan, J., Tantayakom, K., & Laongpech, S. (2014). Efficacy and safety of curcuma domestica extracts compared with ibuprofen in patients with knee osteoarthritis: A multicenter study. *Clinical Interventions in Aging*, 451. https://doi.org/10.2147/cia.s58535

11.Khajehdehi, P., Zanjaninejad, B., Aflaki, E., Nazarinia, M., Azad, F., Malekmakan, L., & Dehghanzadeh, G. (2012). Oral supplementation of turmeric decreases Proteinuria, hematuria, and systolic blood pressure in patients suffering from relapsing or refractory lupus nephritis: A randomized and placebo-controlled study. *Journal of Renal Nutrition*, *22*(1), 50-57. https://doi.org/10.1053/j.jrn.2011.03.002

12.Wu, S. H., Hang, L. W., Yang, J. S., Chen, H. Y., Lin, H. Y., Chiang, J. H., Lu, C. C., Yang, J. L., Lai, T. Y., Ko, Y. C., & Chung, J. G. (2010). Curcumin induces apoptosis in human non-small cell lung cancer NCI-H460 cells through ER stress and caspase cascade- and mitochondria-dependent pathways. *Anticancer research*, *30*(6), 2125–2133.

13.Sharma, R. A., McLelland, H. R., Hill, K. A., Ireson, C. R., Euden, S. A., Manson, M. M., Pirmohamed, M., Marnett, L. J., Gescher, A. J., & Steward, W. P. (2001). Pharmacodynamic and pharmacokinetic study of oral Curcuma extract in patients with colorectal cancer. *Clinical cancer research :*

an official journal of the American Association for Cancer Research, 7(7), 1894–1900.

14.Bläuer, M., Rovio, P. H.,Ylikomi, T., & Heinonen, P. K. (2009). Vitamin D inhibits myometrial and leiomyoma cell proliferation in vitro. *Fertility and Sterility, 91*(5), 1919-1925. https://doi.org/10.1016/j.fertnstert.2008.02.136

15.Baird, D. D., Hill, M. C., Schectman, J. M., & Hollis, B. W. (2013). Vitamin D and the risk of uterine fibroids. *Epidemiology, 24*(3), 447- 453. https://doi.org/10.1097/ede.0b013e31828acca0

16.Munger, K. L., Levin, L. I., Hollis, B. W., Howard, N. S., & Ascherio, A. (2006). Serum 25-Hydroxyvitamin D levels and risk of multiple sclerosis. *JAMA, 296*(23), 2832. https://doi.org/10.1001/jama.296.23.2832

17.Judd, S. E., & Tangpricha, V. (2009). Vitamin D deficiency and risk for cardiovascular disease. *The American Journal of the Medical Sciences, 338*(1), 40-44. https://doi.org/10.1097/maj.0b013e3181aaee91

18.Urashima, M., Segawa, T., Okazaki, M., Kurihara, M., Wada, Y., & Ida, H. (2010). Randomized trial of vitamin D supplementation to prevent seasonal influenza A in schoolchildren. *The American Journal of Clinical Nutrition, 91*(5), 1255-1260. https://doi.org/10.3945/ajcn.2009.29094

19.Al-Hendy, A., Roshdy, Rajaratnam, Maitra, Sabry, M., & Ait Allah. (2013). Treatment of symptomatic uterine fibroids with green tea extract: A pilot randomized controlled clinical study. *International Journal of Women's Health*, 477. https://doi.org/10.2147/ijwh.s41021

20.Eng, Q. Y., Thanikachalam, P. V., & Ramamurthy, S. (2018). Molecular understanding of Epigallocatechin gallate (EGCG) in cardiovascular and metabolic diseases. *Journal of Ethnopharmacology, 210*, 296-310. https://doi.org/10.1016/j.jep.2017.08.035

21.Adaji, S. E., Bature, S. B., & Shittu, O. S. (2012). Vaginally inserted herbs causing vesico-vaginal fistula and vaginal stenosis. *International Urogynecology Journal, 24*(6), 1057-1058. https://doi.org/10.1007/s00192-012-1879-8

22.Chiaffarino, F. (1999). Diet and uterine myomas. *Obstetrics & Gynecology, 94*(3), 395-398. https://doi.org/10.1016/s0029-7844(99)00305-1

23.Wise, L. A., Radin, R. G., Kumanyika, S. K., Ruiz-Narváez, E. A., Palmer, J. R., & Rosenberg, L. (2014). Prospective study of dietary fat and risk of uterine leiomyomata. *The American Journal of Clinical Nutrition, 99*(5), 1105-1116. https://doi.org/10.3945/ajcn.113.073635

24.DuBois, C. M., Beach, S. R., Kashdan, T. B., Nyer, M. B., Park, E. R., Celano, C. M., & Huffman, J. C. (2012). Positive psychological attributes and cardiac outcomes: Associations, mechanisms, and interventions. *Psychosomatics, 53*(4), 303-318. https://doi.org/10.1016/j.psym.2012.04.004

25.Rasmussen, H. N., Scheier, M. F., & Greenhouse, J. B.

(2009). Optimism and physical health: A meta-analytic review. *Annals of Behavioral Medicine, 37*(3), 239-256. https://doi.org/10.1007/s12160-009-9111-x

26.Tindle, H. A., Chang, Y., Kuller, L. H., Manson, J. E., Robinson, J. G., Rosal, M. C., Siegle, G. J., & Matthews, K. A. (2009). Optimism, cynical hostility, and incident coronary heart disease and mortality in the women's health initiative. *Circulation, 120*(8), 656-662. https://doi.org/10.1161/circulationaha.108.827642

27.Brydon, L., Walker, C., Wawrzyniak, A. J., Chart, H., & Steptoe, A. (2009). Dispositional optimism and stress-induced changes in immunity and negative mood. *Brain, Behavior, and Immunity, 23*(6), 810-816. https://doi.org/10.1016/j.bbi.2009.02.018

28.Baird, D. D., Dunson, D. B., Hill, M. C., Cousins, D., & Schectman, J. M. (2006). Association of physical activity with development of uterine Leiomyoma. *American Journal of Epidemiology, 165*(2), 157-163. https://doi.org/10.1093/aje/kwj363

Made in the USA
Monee, IL
04 November 2026

67377461R00030